# OGADEN HORSE

## The Complete Handbook on How To Raising And Caring For Ogaden Horse

## CHAD BRUNO

Table of Contents

## Introductory

The Ogaden region, which spans eastern Ethiopia, Somalia, and Djibouti, is the birthplace of the Ogaden horse, also known as the Somali pony. It's a small, compact horse with special adaptations for the harsh climate and terrain of its native land.

• Ogaden horses are well-known for their toughness, stamina, and resilience in the face of adversity. In the dry and semi-arid regions of East Africa, they are commonly utilized as workhorses, primarily for jobs like herding livestock, as well as for riding and transportation. Because of their stamina and toughness, these horses are ideal for lengthy travels over rough terrain.

• Despite its diminutive stature—typically between 12 and 13 hands (48 and 52 inches)—the breed is highly respected for its speed, agility, and adaptability in its natural habitat. Ogaden horses can be identified by their elegant head, straight profile, and proportionate physique. Gray is one of the more prevalent coat colors, though there are others.

Particularly among the Somali and Oromo peoples, the Ogaden horse is vital to traditional culture and economic survival. It is an integral element of the local culture and has been for generations due to its usefulness in transportation and herding.

• There have been efforts to safeguard and maintain the Ogaden horse because of the threats it faces, such as hybridization with other horse breeds and shifts in land usage. There have been conservation efforts launched to ensure the survival of this rare breed and its cultural significance.

# CHAPTER ONE
## How to Choose an Ogaden Horse

Careful deliberation is required while selecting an Ogaden horse, as with any other breed, to guarantee a healthy and suitable mount. When choosing an Ogaden horse, it is important to keep in mind the following:

**1.** The goal is to find out what the horse will be used for. Which type of horse—one used for herding or transportation, one used for riding, or one kept as a pet—are you interested in? Your decision should be based on your individual requirements.

**2.** Examine the horse for indicators of health and correct conformation. Keep an eye out for a square jaw, a solid chest, strong legs, and symmetrical features. The horse shouldn't have any visible health problems like lameness.

**3.** Evaluate the horse's disposition. Horses from the Ogaden region are well-known for their versatility and pleasant demeanor. It will be much simpler to train a horse that is relaxed and cooperative.

**4.** Think about how old your horse is. Younger horses may require more instruction and time to mature, whereas older horses may have more experience but could also have more wear and strain on their bodies.

**5**. Learn as much as you can about the horse's background and training. Find out if the horse is well-handled, if it knows the tasks you intend to give it, and if it has been schooled for your specific goal.

**6.** Spend some time with the horse and observe its demeanor and reaction. Check out its behavior when exposed to different people. You can learn about its character and whether or not it will cooperate with humans from this.

**7. Pedigree:** If you're interested in breeding or the horse's lineage, inquire about its pedigree. The history and pedigree of a horse can be learned via its breeding papers.

**8.** Inquire with the current owner about the horse's medical and behavioral history, as well as any incidents in which the horse was injured or ill. Knowing the history of the horse can help riders better appreciate him.

**9. Examination by a Veterinarian:** A thorough evaluation of the horse's health and soundness should be performed prior to purchase. X-rays and other diagnostic procedures could fall under this category.

**10.** Consider your financial constraints and shop around for the best deal on an Ogaden horse. Age, training, pedigree, and general quality can all affect the asking price.

**11.** In terms of the law, you should make sure that your ownership documents and health certificates are in order.

**12.** Consult an experienced horse professional, trainer, or veterinarian if you lack the knowledge necessary to choose a horse.

It's important to take your time and do your research when choosing an Ogaden horse because you'll be working with him or her for a long time.

## Stabling and Infrastructure for Horses

In order to maintain a safe, comfortable, and healthy environment for horses, proper housing and facilities are required. The health of the horses and the effectiveness of horse-related management are both enhanced by suitable housing and facilities.

When planning for horse housing and facilities, keep in mind the following:

**1. Stabling:** Stables are essential in areas with extreme weather because they provide shelter for horses. It's important to give each horse sufficient space, natural light, and ventilation when building a stable. The health and well-being of the horse depends on the stall's adequate size and construction.

**2.** Horses need pastures or paddocks where they can run around, graze, and interact with other horses. In order to prevent overgrazing, pastures should be large enough and of high enough quality to meet the needs of the horses and be rotated regularly.

**3.** Secure, equine-friendly fencing is essential for keeping horses safe and preventing them from escaping. Wooden rail, post and rail, vinyl, and electric fencing are all common choices for enclosing a horse's pasture.

**4. Amenities:** Include amenities such as water troughs, feeders, and shelters in pastures and paddocks to ensure horses have access to food, water, and protection from the elements.

**5.** Barns and facilities should have wide aisles and walkways for easy horse and equipment transportation. Slip-resistant flooring should be installed in high-risk areas.

**6.** Saddles, bridles, and other riding gear require a designated space called a "tack room." Maintain a safe, well-ventilated, and well-organized tack room.

**7.** Bathing and grooming horses, particularly after a workout, calls for the use of a special wash rack equipped with both hot and cold running water.

**8.** Maintain a clean and sanitary environment for the horses and their caregivers by instituting a system for the collection, transportation, and disposal of manure.

**9.** Hay, feed, bedding, and equipment must be stored in a way that keeps them dry, organized, and pest-free.

**10.** To train, exercise, and ride horses, you might want to set up an arena or riding area. These spots could be anywhere, indoors or out, depending on the weather and your preferences.

**11**. Protect the building from theft and trespassers by making sure it is locked down tight. The well-being of the horses and the tools relies on this.

**12**. Install fire extinguishers, smoke detectors, and means of egress in all stables and other buildings.

**13**. Keep the stables and pastures stocked with clean, fresh water at all times for optimal hydration. In chilly regions, it may be necessary to use heated water sources.

**14.** Horses and their caregivers need good lighting for their safety, especially when they are feeding, grooming, or performing other routine daily tasks.

**15.** Horses can develop respiratory problems if the air quality in their stables and barns isn't properly maintained through ventilation. This can be accomplished through the use of fans and open windows.

When designing horse housing and facilities, it is crucial to take into account the unique requirements of your horses as well as the local climate. The facilities must be well-maintained and regularly inspected to guarantee they continue to accommodate the horses' needs.

Horses need a well-balanced diet to thrive physically and mentally, which in turn improves their performance. Horses' nutritional needs can vary based on factors like age, activity level, breed, and individual health. **The following are some suggested feeding practices and diets for horses:**

## 1. Grass and hay for livestock:

• High-quality forage, such as grass hay (e.g., timothy, bermudagrass, or orchardgrass) or legume hay (e.g., alfalfa or clover), should form the basis of a horse's diet. Forage should be available to horses at all times.

• Pasture is a great place to get your forage, but it needs to be managed properly to avoid overgrazing and weight gain.

## 2. Grain Concentrates:

• Concentrates, such as grains (e.g., oats, corn, barley), and commercial feeds, can be added to the diet to boost energy and supplement deficiencies.

• Concentrates should be fed in amounts determined by the individual horse's nutritional requirements. Don't stuff yourself, as this can lead to weight gain and metabolic problems.

## 3. Protein:

Protein is essential for horses because it helps them build and repair muscle. Good sources of protein include alfalfa hay, soybean meal, and commercial feeds.

• The horse's age and level of activity will determine the optimal protein content of the diet.

## 4. Minerals and Vitamins:

• Make sure you're getting enough of the nutrients you need every day. These are commonly found in commercially available horse feed. If not, you might want to think about taking a supplement.

Horses should have access to salt blocks so they can control their salt intake.

## 5. Water:

• Maintain a constant supply of fresh water for your horse. It's important to drink enough water because dehydration can cause a host of medical issues.

## 6. How Often They Eat:

• Horses have small stomachs and are meant to graze continuously. If you can, try to emulate their natural feeding pattern by giving them several short meals throughout the day.

## 7. Evaluation of Physical Health:

• Use a body condition score scale on a regular basis to evaluate your horse's health. If necessary, make dietary changes to keep the body in peak shape.

## 8. Food Restrictions:

• Due to their health or level of exercise, certain horses have unique nutritional requirements. For advice on specific diets, speak with your vet or an equine nutritionist.

## 9. Don't Pile On The Pounds

• Obesity and its related health issues are a direct result of overfeeding. The ideal weight for a horse depends on its age, breed, and degree of exercise.

## 10. Check on Your Teeth's Health:

• Check the health of your horse's teeth regularly. If they have dental problems, they may have trouble chewing and digesting their food.

## 11. Avoid Sudden Changes in Your Diet:

• Altering the horse's food should be done gradually to avoid causing stomach problems. The digestive tracts of horses are quite delicate.

## 12. Needs Unique to Horses:

• Take into account the varying requirements of various horse types, such as young horses, mares in various stages of pregnancy and lactation, older horses, and horses used for labor. It's possible that they need a change in nutrition as a result.

## 13. Exercising and Being Active:

• A horse's nutritional needs may vary depending on the type and quantity of work it is expected to perform. Horses that perform extensive work may require extra food and water.

It's crucial to speak with an equine nutritionist or veterinarian to design a feeding plan that is suited to your horse's individual needs. Keep in mind that each horse has its own set of nutritional needs, so it's important to monitor their overall health and well-being on a regular basis.

## CHAPTER TWO
### Medicine and Animals

Keeping your horse in good shape and getting him regular veterinary care is crucial to his happiness and longevity. Some fundamentals of horse health and veterinary medicine are as follows:

## 1. Routine checkups:

• Have your horse examined regularly by a licensed veterinarian who specializes in horses. Physical exams, dental exams, and immunizations are all part of these checkups.

## 2. Vaccinations:

• Talk to your vet about creating a vaccine regimen that takes into account your horse's age, where you live, and how often you ride. Diseases including tetanus, rabies, West Nile virus, and equine influenza all have vaccines that protect against them.

## 3. Deworming:

• Work with your vet to create a deworming schedule for effective internal parasite management. Your horse's deworming schedule and regimen should be designed just for him.

## 4. Oral Health:

• Proper chewing and digestion rely on regular dental checkups and floating (file down sharp points and uneven surfaces).

## 5. Care for Horses' Hooves:

• Maintaining healthy hooves requires regular care, such as trimming and shoeing. In addition, it aids in the avoidance of lameness and other foot problems.

## 6. Nutrition:

• Develop a healthy diet plan tailored to your horse's requirements with the help of a professional equine nutritionist. Health and productivity greatly benefit from eating right.

## 7. Evaluation of Physical Health:

• Use a body condition rating system on a regular basis to evaluate your horse's health. Maintain a healthy weight by making the necessary changes to one's diet and exercise routine.

## 8. Exercise:

• To keep your horse in good shape physically and mentally, it is important to provide it frequent exercise.

## 9. Elimination of Pests:

• Control external parasites (such as flies and ticks) with tools including fly sprays, fly sheets, and protective footwear.

## 10. Ecological Safety:

• Make sure the stable is spotless, secure, and devoid of any potential dangers for the horse. This entails doing things like keeping pests at bay and managing manure.

## 11. Being Ready for an Emergency:

• Warning! Equine Emergencies Must Be Prepared For! Be prepared for emergencies by always carrying a first aid kit and learning how to treat the most frequent ailments. Your pet's vet should be able to help.

## 12. Immunization Documents:

• Document all of your horse's medical care, including vaccinations, deworming, and more. You'll need this data to keep track of your horse's medical history.

## 13. Male Sterilization and Birth Control:

• If you don't want to use your stallions or mares for breeding, you may choose to regulate their reproduction or have them castrated.

## 14. Moderate and frequent physical activity:

• Exercising regularly is essential for a healthy body, active mind, and fulfilling social life. Having access to a pasture or paddock on a regular basis is ideal.

## 15. Travel Factors to Consider:
The stress and health dangers of transporting a horse should be taken into account. During trips, make sure the horse has plenty of water and rests.

## 16. Training and Behaviour:

• Deal with any training or behavioral concerns through appropriate training, and get expert help if needed.

## 17. Equine Seniors and Those with Special Needs:

• Horses in their twilight years or with particular needs require special treatment. For advice on issues relating to old age, see your vet.

Keep in mind that your horse is an individual with special requirements; therefore, it is essential to collaborate closely with your veterinarian and other equine professionals to create a thorough healthcare plan. A long and healthy life for your horse is possible with the help of preventative medicine and early diagnosis and treatment of any health problems.

## Methods for a Nice Haircut

Your horse's health and attractiveness depend on regular grooming. Grooming your horse regularly has several benefits, including keeping it clean and comfortable and detecting injuries, skin disorders, and other health problems. Here are some essential tips and procedures for personal grooming:

**1. Tying the Horse Up or Restraining It:**

• Put the horse in a secure area, such as a grooming stall or cross ties, or use a quick-release knot.

**2. Cavalry Hoof Care:**

• Hoof picking should be the first step. Clean the sole and frog of any mud, gravel, or other debris. Examine the hooves for thrush or any other symptoms of damage.

### 3. Cleaning and Dusting:

• Use a curry comb in a circular motion to remove debris and stray hair first. Use caution so as not to irritate the other person. Follow the direction of your hair's natural development.

• Use a stiff brush (a body brush or a dandy brush) to remove the dirt and hair that has been loosened.

To ensure a glossy, smooth finish, use a light brush to apply the last coat. Make sure you give your face and legs the care they need.

## 4. Coat and Tail Maintenance:

• Detangle the mane and tail and brush out any debris with a wide-toothed comb or dedicated mane and tail brush.

• Horses with long manes and tails may benefit from a detangler or conditioner, so use it if necessary.

Avoid ripping or tearing the hair by being careful.

## 5. Cleaning Your Face:

• Wipe the horse's eyes, nose, and muzzle with a damp sponge or towel. Take care not to irritate the delicate skin around your eyes.

- Look for evidence of nasal or ocular discharge.

## 6. Cleaning Your Ears

- Use a soft, wet cloth or a specialized ear-cleaning product to gently wipe the inside of the horse's ears. Be careful not to push material farther into the ear.

## 7. Trimming (If Desired):

- Clippers can be used to remove excess hair from the body, face, and other regions of your horse. To prevent skin irritation, keep the blades sharp and tidy.

**8. Occasional Bathing:**

• A thorough horse bath may be required if the animal is particularly grimy. Wash the horse using a gentle sponge or brush and a pail of warm water containing horse shampoo. Thoroughly rinsing and drying the horse with a clean cooler or cloth is required.

**9. Inspect for Abnormalities and Injuries:**

• Look for wounds, rashes, lumps, or other symptoms of illness while grooming the horse. Pay attention to changes in the skin, such as rashes or swelling.

**10.** Braiding the tail is an alternative way to maintain it neat and tangle-free. This is routine in competitive and display situations.

**11.** To take care of your horse's feet, try using a hoof conditioner or dressing. Examine the hooves for splits, damage, and other problems.

**12.** Use fly spray or other insect repellents to keep flies and other pests off the horse as you groom him.

**13.** Use grooming as a positive reinforcement chance to connect with your horse. Make the experience fun for the horse by being patient and offering goodies or positive reinforcement.

In addition to promoting the well-being and aesthetics of your horse, regular grooming sessions also give you the chance to forge a close emotional connection with your animal friend. You and your horse should look forward to grooming sessions.

## CHAPTER THREE
### Different Exercise Routines for Various Purposes

Horses need to be exercised in a way that is appropriate for their age, fitness level, discipline, and individual goals. It is important to personalize the workout to the specific demands of your horse and your goals. Here are some examples of workout plans tailored to specific needs:

## 1. Preventative Medicine and Wellness:

• Objective: Preserve physical and mental well-being.

Turn out your horse often in a pasture or paddock so he can exercise and socialize in his natural environment. To maintain your horse's health and happiness, try some easy rides or groundwork.

## 2. Obesity and weight loss management:

• The purpose of this project is to assist overweight horses in losing weight and keeping it off.

• **Plan:** Include both walking and aerobic exercise (trotting, cantering) and gradually increase the intensity and length. Keep an eye on your dietary intake to make sure you're getting enough of the right nutrients and not too much.

## 3. Gaining Muscle and Stamina:

• Targeted muscle group training for enhanced performance.

Hill work, pole work, and lunges are all great examples of workouts to add to your routine. Develop your muscles just as your trainer instructs you to by engaging in regular, systematic exercise.

## 4. Perseverance and Energy:

• Objective: Improve the horse's endurance so that it can be used for longer rides, trail riding, or races.

- **Plan:** Work up to longer and harder workouts over time. Incorporate LSD rides or trot sets to increase stamina and endurance. Injury can be avoided with moderate conditioning.

## 5. Dressage, or the Art of Exact Rides:

- Flexibility, equilibrium, and accuracy are developed for use in dressage and other precision sports.

- **Routine:** Regular, low-impact exercise is emphasized. Practice flexibility by moving laterally, making smooth transitions, and stretching. Flexibility and correct form should be prioritized.

## 6. Event Jumping:

• Improve the horse's overall jumping performance by working on its speed and power.

Jumping technique can be enhanced with a regular routine that includes gymnastic exercises and gridwork. Exercises like cavaletti and brief leaps on the pole can help you gain strength and stability.

## 7. Eventing:

• The objective is to train for events that include all three disciplines of eventing: dressage, cross-country, and show jumping.

To create a well-rounded athlete, a program should include dressage work, jumping drills, and cross-country running. To improve stamina, do hill sprints and gallop.

**8. Racing:**

• **Purpose:** Get in shape to run either a flat race or a steeplechase.

• **Routine:** Carry out targeted workouts that improve your speed and cardiovascular health. Sprints, gallops, and interval training are common components.

## 9. Healing and Recuperation:

Help a horse get well after it's been hurt or has surgery.

• **Routine:** Collaborate closely with your veterinarian to develop a tailored rehabilitation program that may include supervised physical activity and therapeutic massage. To speed up recovery without re-injuring yourself, it's best to move slowly and deliberately.

**10.** The purpose of senior horse care is to ensure the continued well-being and comfort of geriatric equines. Provide a routine that includes light riding and walking on a regular basis. Provide joint supplements as indicated by a veterinarian, and create a comfortable living environment.

Maintaining the horse's physical and mental health is your top priority, so it's important to keep tabs on the animal's condition, make adjustments to its exercise routine as needed, and talk to a vet, trainer, or equestrian specialist for advice. All equine exercise programs should prioritize safety, consistency, and progressive overload.

Horse breeding is a serious endeavor that calls for forethought, expertise, and moral deliberation. It's crucial to have a firm grasp on the following points and procedures before beginning a breeding program:

## 1. Breeding Programs:

• Pick out potential mares and stallions that meet your needs in terms of breed, conformation, health, temperament, and performance. Think about what you hope to achieve with your breeding program and make sure the two of you are a good genetic match.

## 2. Evaluation of Health:

• Make sure the mare and the stallions are both in tip-top shape. Veterinarian checkups, immunizations, deworming, and dental treatment are all part of this routine.

## 3. Testing for Optimal Procreation:

• Ensure the fertility of the mare and stallion by having them tested for reproductive health.

## 4. Methods of Breeding:

• The first step in breeding is deciding whether to use artificial insemination (AI) or natural mating (live cover). Artificial intelligence (AI) provides for increased management and the potential usage of stallions that are not physically present.

## 5. Timing:

• When it comes to breeding, timing is everything. Determine the best time to breed by keeping track of the mare's estrus cycle and ovulation.

## 6. Confirmation of Pregnancy:

• After a successful mating, you should check the pregnant mare with an ultrasound or a veterinarian inspection.

## 7. Antenatal Care:

• Pregnant mares need a healthy diet, regular exercise, and immunizations to ensure a healthy pregnancy and baby. A veterinarian should be consulted for individualized treatment options.

## 8. Ahead of the Foaling:

• Make sure the foaling place is clean and secure. Prepare it for the new arrival by stocking it with fresh linens, towels, and a foaling kit.

## 9. Help with Foaling:

• Always be prepared to lend a hand if requested during the foaling process. Keep an eye on the mare for any symptoms of trouble.

**10.** After the foal is born, the mare and foal should be given the proper postpartum care, which includes giving the foal colostrum, caring for the umbilical cord, and taking the foal to the veterinarian.

**11.** Foals benefit greatly from being handled and socialized from an early age to help them adjust to life among humans.

**12**. Foal registration and identity documents (passport, microchip) should be obtained from the relevant breed organization.

**13.** Think about the moral consequences of breeding, such as your accountability for the safety of the stallions, mares, and offspring. Always be willing to take on the responsibilities of a lifetime caretaker.

**14.** Genetics and Horse Health: Learn about horse ancestry and heritable characteristics so you can pick the best offspring. Potential health problems passed down via families can be discovered with genetic testing.

**15.** Research the current and potential demand for the breed of horse you intend to breed. Make sure there is a customer base for your foals.

**16.** Make sure foals only go to responsible, caring homes where they will receive the attention and care they need.

**17. Legal Matters:** - Be familiar with and abide by all applicable local, state, and federal laws pertaining to horse breeding, including those governing registration, transportation, and animal welfare.

Responsible breeding is not something to be taken lightly because it requires dedication to the animals' well-being. Only when there is a well-defined goal and an approach to the horses' welfare may breeding be pursued. Throughout the breeding process, advice from horse experts, doctors, and breed associations can be invaluable.

## Methods and Disciplines of Horseback Riding

In the equestrian realm, there is a broad variety of riding techniques and disciplines, each with its own distinct set of abilities, equipment, and aims. The most widely practiced forms of riding are as follows:

## 1. Riding in England:

• An English rider uses both hands on the reins and sits in a close-contact saddle. There are several fields that fall under its umbrella.

Dressage is the practice of teaching a horse to perform a complex series of maneuvers with precision and balance.

• Show Jumping is a timed sport in which riders guide their horses over a series of hurdles.

Eventing is a triathlon that includes dressage, cross-country, and show jumping.

Hunt Seat Equitation, which is commonly seen in equitation classes, places an emphasis on the rider's form and elegance.

## 2. Regions West:

• The Western saddle and one-handed rein control are hallmarks of the Western riding style. It encompasses fields such as:

• Reining is a pattern-based competition in which the horse spins, slides, and executes other elaborate moves.

Cutting is a type of horsemanship in which riders demonstrate their mounts' intelligence by separating a single cow from a herd.

• Western Pleasure: Emphasizes the fluidity of the horse's gaits and a relaxed, responsive disposition.

### 3. Riding the Trails:

• Trail riding is a type of recreational riding in which riders traverse undeveloped landscapes, forests, and trails at their own pace.

**4.** Endurance riding is distinguished by its emphasis on long distance travel, often between 50 and 100 miles each day. Horse and rider stamina and conditioning are paramount.

### 5. Polo:

• Polo is a team sport performed on horseback, with riders using mallets to score goals by smashing a ball into the other team's goal.

## 6. The Rodeo:

• The term "rodeo" is used to describe a variety of Western-style competitions, such as bull riding, saddle bronc riding, bareback bronc riding, and steer wrestling.

## 7. Vaulting:

• To demonstrate agility, strength, and coordination, vaulters perform gymnastic and dance routines while riding a moving horse.

## 8. In a Saddle:

• The American Saddle bred and other high-stepping horse breeds are ideal for saddle seat riding because of their high-stepping gaits.

## 9. Driving a Carriage:

• Driving a carriage or cart pulled by a horse or team of horses is called carriage driving. There are a wide variety of driving competitions, from leisure to combined.

**10. Mounted Games:** - Mounted games are equestrian competitions that place a premium on riding skill, speed, and agility.

**11.** Individuals with impairments can benefit greatly from therapeutic riding, which use horseback riding as a method of physical, occupational, and emotional treatment.

**12.** In horse ball, riders try to score goals by kicking a ball into a basket attached to their horse's saddle.

**13**. Riding a horse across a course full of natural obstacles is known as "cross-country," and it's one of the many eventing disciplines.

**14.** Using both reining and cutting techniques, riders in the Western riding discipline of reined cow horse work cattle.

Different riding styles and disciplines call for different

abilities, education, and gear. The ambitions and interests of riders, as well as the natural talents and training of their horses, often lead them to focus on one or more distinct disciplines. To ensure one's own safety and success in any of these fields, one must first acquire suitable instruction and supervision from qualified instructors.

## CHAPTER FOUR
### The Good and the Right

Horse ownership, training, and care that prioritize the animal's well-being is considered responsible. Protecting horses from unethical treatment is not just the right thing to do, but also the law in many places. Some fundamental ethical concepts concerning the well-being of horses are as follows:

## 1. Legal Possession:

• Ethical horse ownership requires a clean, healthy environment free from hazards for the horses. Horses rely on their owners to meet their physiological, psychological, and behavioral requirements.

## 2. Life satisfaction:

• Horses need regular access to fresh water and a well-balanced food. They need to be shielded from the elements and given refuge if it becomes necessary.

## 3. Medical Care:

• Regular veterinary treatment is vital to maintain a horse's health and well-being. Vaccinations, dental work, deworming, and medical attention for injuries and illnesses all fall under this category.

## 4. Proper Instruction:

• Only employ positive reinforcement and treat the horse with kindness and courtesy during training. Don't resort to harmful measures like physical violence or intimidating tactics.

## 5. Keeping From Burning Out:

• Horses shouldn't be overworked or put through strenuous physical activities. Preventing weariness and injury requires enough rest and recuperation.

## 6. Checking the Health of a Subject:

• Check the horse's condition frequently and make dietary and activity changes as needed. Avoid either overfeeding or underfeeding your horse, as either is detrimental to its health.

## 7. Reproductive Ethics:

• Responsible breeding takes into account the genetic history, physical condition, and emotional well-being of both the mare and the stallion. It's best not to breed too many animals or those who have a history of certain diseases.

## 8. Effects on the Environment:

• The ecological effects of horse ownership should be taken into account. Reduce environmental damage through proper waste management, manure disposal, and land application.

## 9. Kindness at the End of Life:

• When deciding whether or not to euthanize a horse, the animal's comfort and quality of life should be taken into account. A qualified veterinarian is the best choice to compassionately put an animal to sleep.

**10.** Compete fairly and honorably in equestrian competitions and other activities. Stay away from illegal substances and unsafe training methods.

**11. Knowledge and Understanding:** - Keep learning about the proper treatment, handling, and ethics of horses. Inform your neighbors and advocate for the well-being of horses and appropriate horse ownership.

**12. Advocacy:** Speak up for the rights of horses locally, nationally, and globally. Please back efforts to improve the lives of horses.

**13.** Maintain conformity with all applicable federal, state, and local animal welfare statutes and regulations. Don't hesitate to contact the police if you suspect neglect or abuse.

**14.** Realize that caring for a horse is a lifelong responsibility. Having a horse requires a significant time commitment and financial investment.

Maintaining the health of horses relies heavily on ethical issues and equine wellbeing. For the duration of their lives, responsible horse owners and professionals will put the horse's well-being ahead of anything else.

## Conclusion

In order to keep these amazing animals healthy, happy, and in good hands, proper horse ownership, care, and management require a wide range of considerations and practices. An in-depth knowledge of equine needs and a dedication to their health are essential in areas ranging from proper feeding and grooming skills to ethical treatment of horses and responsible breeding practices. No matter how much or how little experience you have with horses, you should always keep the fundamentals of equine care, training, and ethics in mind.

You can keep your horse healthy and avoid common problems by giving it the right food, exercise, and shelter, and by taking it to the vet regularly. In addition to enhancing the horse's behavior and performance, ethical training and handling approaches also fortify the partnership between horse and rider.

Your goals and the horse's ability will determine whether you ride English or Western, and you should always consider the horse's comfort and well-being when making this decision. If breeding is to be done, it must be done ethically and with careful attention to genetics.

In the end, what matters most is the horses' morality and well-being. Treating horses with respect, care, and consideration is not only a moral requirement but a legal one in many locations. From the time they are foals until they reach their retirement years, all owners, trainers, and enthusiasts of horses have a duty to treat these magnificent animals with the utmost respect and care. Equestrians may protect horses' well-being for the long term and continue to enjoy their company thanks to these guidelines.

**THE END**